ALKALINE

HEALING DIET FOR

BEGINNERS

The Ultimate Guide to Healthy, Quick and Easy Recipes for Natural Weight Loss and Improved Immune System

ANNIE FRANKLIN

TABLE OF CONTENTS

INTRODUCTION   **5**

Chapter One   **10**

Understanding the Alkaline Vegan Healing Diet   **10**

1.1 What is an Alkaline Vegan Diet?   10

1.2 The Healing Power of Alkaline Foods   11

1.3 Benefits of Adopting an Alkaline Vegan Diet   13

1.4 How the Alkaline Diet Supports Natural Weight Loss   15

1.5 Strengthening Your Immune System with Alkaline Foods   17

Chapter Two   **20**

Getting Started with the Alkaline Vegan Healing Diet   **20**

2.1 Setting the Right Mindset for Success   20

2.2 Grocery Shopping for Alkaline
Vegan Ingredients   21

2.3 Stocking Your Alkaline Vegan
Pantry   22

2.4 Meal Planning for Optimal
Results   23

2.5 Tips for Dining Out on the
Alkaline Vegan Diet   24

Chapter Three   **26**

Energizing Breakfast Recipes **26**

3.1 Energizing Green Smoothie
Bowl   26

3.2 Alkaline Chia Seed Pudding   28

3.3 Zesty Citrus Avocado Toast   30

Chapter Four   **33**

Nutrient-Rich Lunchtime Delights 33

4.1 Rainbow Veggie Quinoa Salad
33

4.2 Creamy Alkaline Gazpacho
Soup   35

4.3 Mediterranean Stuffed Bell Peppers   37

Chapter Five   **41**

Nourishing Dinner Options   **41**

5.1 Baked Portobello Mushrooms with Garlic Kale   41

5.2 Coconut Curry Lentil Stew   43

5.3 Roasted Cauliflower Steaks with Tahini Dressing   46

Chapter Six   **49**

Tasty Snacks to Satisfy Cravings   **49**

6.1 Alkaline Trail Mix   49

6.2 Baked Zucchini Chips with Cashew Dip   51

6.3 Refreshing Cucumber and Watermelon Salad   54

Chapter Seven   **56**

Indulgent Desserts with a Healthy Twist   **56**

7.1 Decadent Almond Butter and

Banana Nice Cream   56

7.2 Raw Vegan Lemon Bars   58

7.3 Guilt-Free Chocolate Avocado
Mousse   61

Chapter Eight   63

**Incorporating Superfoods into Your
Alkaline Vegan Diet   63**

8.1 Exploring the Power of
Superfoods   63

8.2 Acai Berry Bowl with Alkaline
Fruits   64

8.3 Spirulina-infused Green
Smoothie   66

Chapter Nine   69

Hydration and Detoxification   69

9.1 Importance of Hydration on an
Alkaline Vegan Diet   69

9.2 Detoxifying Lemon Ginger
Water   71

9.3 Refreshing Cucumber and Mint

Detox Drink   73

Chapter Ten   **76**

**Creating Balance and Sustainable
Habits**   **76**

10.1 Balancing Alkaline Vegan Diet
with Other Lifestyle Factors   77

10.2 Tips for Long-term Success 79

10.3 Staying Motivated on Your
Healing Journey   81

**Embracing the Alkaline Vegan
Healing Diet for Life**   **84**

BONUS   **89**

Alkaline Vegan Healing Food List
89

28-day meal plan for the Alkaline
Vegan Healing Diet   95

INTRODUCTION

The Alkaline Vegan Diet finds its roots in two fundamental principles: alkalinity and plant-based nutrition. The concept of alkalinity dates back to ancient civilizations, where traditional healers and philosophers recognized the importance of maintaining a balanced pH level in the body for optimal health. Alkaline-forming foods were believed to have a positive effect on the body's internal environment, promoting healing and overall well-being.

The modern Alkaline Vegan Diet was popularized by Dr. Sebi (Alfredo Darrington Bowman), a renowned herbalist and natural healer. Dr. Sebi devoted his life to studying the relationship between food and health and believed that the human body thrives best in an alkaline state. He advocated for a plant-based diet consisting of foods that are naturally alkaline, avoiding highly acidic and processed foods. Dr. Sebi's teachings gained significant attention and inspired countless individuals to adopt the Alkaline Vegan Diet as a means to transform their health.

Convincing Truths for Consideration

1. **Scientific Research:** While the Alkaline Vegan Diet may have historical roots, modern scientific research increasingly supports the health benefits of plant-based diets. Numerous studies have shown that a diet rich in fruits, vegetables, nuts, and seeds is associated with a lower risk of chronic diseases and improved overall health.

2. **Sustainable and Environmentally Friendly:** Choosing a plant-based diet is not only beneficial for personal health but also for the planet. The production of plant-based foods generally requires fewer resources and generates fewer greenhouse gas emissions compared to animal-based products, making it a more sustainable and environmentally friendly choice.

3. **Personal Testimonials:** Countless individuals have shared their transformative experiences with the Alkaline Vegan Diet, recounting improvements in their health, energy levels, and overall well-being. These testimonials highlight the real-life impact that this dietary approach can have on people's lives.

4. **Emphasis on Whole Foods:** The Alkaline Vegan Diet encourages the consumption of whole, unprocessed foods, which aligns with what many nutrition experts advocate. This focus on whole foods ensures that individuals obtain essential nutrients and antioxidants that are crucial for optimal health.

5. **Customizable and Flexible:** The Alkaline Vegan Diet can be adapted to various preferences and dietary restrictions. With a wide variety of plant-based ingredients available, individuals can personalize their meals to suit their tastes and needs while still enjoying the benefits of this dietary approach.

The Alkaline Vegan Diet is not just a passing trend but a time-tested and scientifically supported approach to nourishing the body, mind, and soul. Its focus on alkalinity and plant-based nutrition offers an array of health benefits, ranging from improved digestion and natural weight loss to enhanced immune function and increased energy. Considering the growing body of evidence and the countless personal success stories, embracing the Alkaline Vegan Diet may prove to be a transformative journey toward a healthier and more vibrant life.

Chapter One

Understanding the Alkaline Vegan Healing Diet

1.1 What is an Alkaline Vegan Diet?

The Alkaline Vegan Diet is a nutritional approach that focuses on consuming plant-based foods that promote a more alkaline pH level in the body. This diet emphasizes the consumption of fresh fruits, vegetables, nuts, seeds, and legumes while avoiding acidic and processed foods. The concept behind this diet is based on the belief that maintaining a slightly alkaline pH level in the body can promote overall health and well-being.

Generally, acidity and alkalinity are measured on the pH scale, it ranges from 0 to 14. A pH level of 7 is considered neutral, while levels below 7 are acidic, and levels above 7 are alkaline. Proponents of the Alkaline Vegan Diet argue that consuming too many acidic foods can disrupt the body's natural pH balance, leading to various health issues. By adopting this diet, individuals aim to shift their pH balance towards the alkaline side, which is believed to have several health benefits.

1.2 The Healing Power of Alkaline Foods

Alkaline foods are rich in essential vitamins, minerals, and antioxidants, which play a significant role in supporting the body's natural healing processes. These foods are typically nutrient-dense and have anti-inflammatory properties, contributing to reduced inflammation in the body.

When the body maintains an alkaline pH level, it creates an environment that is less conducive to the growth and proliferation of harmful microorganisms. This may lead to improved digestion and better absorption of nutrients, thus supporting the body's ability to heal and repair itself.

Alkaline foods are often associated with improved hydration. Proper hydration is essential for the optimal functioning of bodily systems, as water plays a crucial role in transporting nutrients and eliminating waste products.

1.3 Benefits of Adopting an Alkaline Vegan Diet

Numerous benefits are attributed to adopting an Alkaline Vegan Diet:

a. **Improved Digestive Health:** Alkaline foods are rich in dietary fiber, which aids digestion and supports a healthy gut. This can lead to reduced bloating, constipation, and a decreased risk of gastrointestinal disorders.

b. **Increased Energy Levels:** Alkaline foods provide a steady source of energy due to their nutrient density. They help stabilize blood sugar levels, preventing energy crashes commonly associated with consuming sugary or processed foods.

c. **Enhanced Immune Function:** Alkaline foods are packed with immune-boosting nutrients such as vitamin C and zinc, which help fortify the body's defenses against infections and diseases.

d. **Reduced Risk of Chronic Diseases:** A diet rich in alkaline foods has been linked to a decreased risk of chronic diseases, such as heart disease and certain types of cancer, mainly due to the abundance of antioxidants and anti-inflammatory compounds.

e. **Weight Management:** Alkaline Vegan Diet followers often experience natural weight loss as a result of consuming nutrient-dense, low-calorie foods and avoiding processed and high-calorie options.

1.4 How the Alkaline Diet Supports Natural Weight Loss

The Alkaline Vegan Diet can be beneficial for weight loss due to several reasons:

a. **Reduced Caloric Intake:** Alkaline foods, such as fresh fruits and vegetables, are generally lower in calories than processed and high-fat foods. As a result, individuals tend to consume fewer calories while feeling more satisfied and nourished.

b. **Improved Digestion:** The diet's emphasis on fiber-rich foods supports healthy digestion and regular bowel movements, reducing the chances of bloating and constipation, which can impact weight management.

c. **Enhanced Metabolism:** Some alkaline foods, like citrus fruits, are known to boost metabolism. A more efficient metabolism can aid in burning calories more effectively.

d. **Reduced Cravings:** By avoiding highly processed and sugary foods, individuals may experience reduced cravings for unhealthy snacks, which can contribute to weight gain.

e. **Balanced Hormones:** Consuming nutrient-dense foods can help regulate hormones that control appetite and satiety, promoting a balanced and healthy approach to eating.

1.5 Strengthening Your Immune System with Alkaline Foods

A robust immune system is vital for defending the body against infections and illnesses. Alkaline foods can play a crucial role in strengthening the immune system:

a. **Rich in Antioxidants:** Alkaline foods, especially colorful fruits and vegetables, are packed with antioxidants that combat free radicals in the body. Free radicals can damage cells and weaken the immune system, but antioxidants neutralize them, thus bolstering immunity.

b. **Vitamin C Powerhouses:** Citrus fruits, leafy greens, and bell peppers, commonly found in an alkaline diet, are abundant sources of vitamin C. This essential nutrient supports immune cell function and enhances the body's ability to fight infections.

c. **Alkaline Minerals:** Foods like almonds and leafy greens are rich in alkaline minerals like magnesium and calcium, which contribute to immune system support and overall health.

d. **Reduced Inflammation:** Chronic inflammation can suppress the immune system. Alkaline foods are known for their anti-inflammatory properties, helping to alleviate inflammation and allowing the immune system to function optimally.

e. **Beneficial Gut Microbiota:** Alkaline foods, being rich in fiber, promote a healthy gut environment, fostering the growth of beneficial gut bacteria. A balanced gut microbiome positively influences immune function.

By adopting an Alkaline Vegan Diet and incorporating a wide variety of nutrient-rich foods into daily meals, individuals can harness the healing power of alkaline foods and experience the numerous benefits they offer for overall health, weight management, and a strengthened immune system.

Chapter Two

Getting Started with the Alkaline Vegan Healing Diet

2.1 Setting the Right Mindset for Success

Before embarking on any dietary journey, it is vital to set the right mindset for success. Embrace the idea that this diet is not a short-term fix but a lifestyle change for long-term health benefits. Understand that your body may undergo a detoxification process as you eliminate acidic and processed foods. Patience and perseverance are crucial during this transition phase.

Educate yourself about the principles of the Alkaline Vegan Healing Diet and the benefits it offers. Surround yourself with a support system, whether it be friends, family, or online communities, to stay motivated and share experiences.

2.2 Grocery Shopping for Alkaline Vegan Ingredients

Grocery shopping for the Alkaline Vegan Healing Diet can be an exciting and fulfilling experience. Focus on fresh, organic, and locally sourced produce. Aim to fill your shopping cart with an abundance of alkaline-forming foods, such as leafy greens (spinach, kale, chard), vegetables (broccoli, cucumbers, bell peppers), fruits (avocado, berries, watermelon), and whole grains (quinoa, millet, buckwheat).

Remember to avoid or minimize acidic foods like meat, dairy, processed foods, and refined sugars. Familiarize yourself with alkaline substitutes for common ingredients, such as using almond milk instead of cow's milk or whole-grain flour instead of refined flour.

2.3 Stocking Your Alkaline Vegan Pantry

Building a well-stocked pantry is essential for maintaining the Alkaline Vegan Healing Diet. Keep your pantry equipped with staples like nuts (almonds, walnuts), seeds (chia, flaxseed), legumes (chickpeas, lentils), and healthy oils (coconut oil, olive oil). These items form the foundation of various nutritious and delicious recipes.

Invest in alkaline seasonings and spices like turmeric, garlic, and cayenne pepper to add flavor to your dishes without compromising their alkalinity. Keep a variety of herbal teas and alkaline-approved snacks to curb any cravings and prevent potential fallbacks.

2.4 Meal Planning for Optimal Results

Meal planning is key to maintaining consistency and ensuring a balanced intake of nutrients. Create a weekly meal plan that incorporates a diverse array of alkaline vegan recipes. Prioritize whole foods and experiment with different cooking methods to retain the maximum nutritional value of your meals.

Batch-cooking and prepping ingredients in advance can save time and help you stay on track, especially on busy days. Incorporate a mix of raw and cooked foods to optimize enzyme intake and ensure a variety of flavors and textures.

2.5 Tips for Dining Out on the Alkaline Vegan Diet

Eating out can pose challenges, but with some preparation, you can still adhere to your Alkaline Vegan Healing Diet. Research restaurants beforehand and look for vegan or plant-based options on the menu. Most establishments are willing to accommodate dietary preferences if you communicate your needs politely.

Customize your orders by asking for extra vegetables, salads, or specific ingredient substitutions. Be mindful of hidden acidic ingredients in dressings or sauces, and opt for simple, oil-free dressings whenever possible.

Note: Embarking on the Alkaline Vegan Healing Diet is a transformative journey that requires dedication and an open mindset. By setting the right intentions, understanding the principles, and planning ahead, you can embrace this lifestyle with confidence. Remember that each person's body is unique, so be patient with yourself and allow time for your body to adapt to the positive changes. The Alkaline Vegan Healing Diet offers a path to vibrant health and wellness, helping you thrive in all aspects of life.

Chapter Three

Energizing Breakfast Recipes

Starting your day with a nutritious and alkalizing breakfast can set a positive tone for the rest of the day.

3.1 Energizing Green Smoothie Bowl

Ingredients:
- 1 cup spinach (or kale), washed and chopped
- 1 ripe banana, peeled and sliced
- 1 cup fresh or frozen mixed berries (blueberries, strawberries, or raspberries)
- ½ cucumber, peeled and chopped
- ½ avocado, peeled and pitted
- 1 tablespoon chia seeds

- 1 cup unsweetened almond milk (or any desired plant-based milk)
- 1 tablespoon almond butter (optional for extra creaminess)
- 1 teaspoon spirulina or wheatgrass powder (optional, for an added alkalizing boost)
- Toppings: Fresh berries, sliced kiwi, unsweetened shredded coconut, and a sprinkle of chia seeds.

Instructions:

1. In a high-speed blender, combine spinach (or kale), banana, mixed berries, cucumber, avocado, chia seeds, almond milk, almond butter, and spirulina or wheatgrass powder (if using).

2. Blend on high until smooth and creamy. If the mixture is too thick, you can add more

almond milk to achieve your desired consistency.

3. Turn the green smoothie into a bowl.

4. Top the smoothie with fresh berries, sliced kiwi, unsweetened shredded coconut, and a sprinkle of chia seeds for added texture and nutrition.

5. Enjoy your Energizing Green Smoothie Bowl immediately, while it's fresh and vibrant!

3.2 Alkaline Chia Seed Pudding

Ingredients:

- ¼ cup chia seeds
- 1 cup unsweetened almond milk (could be any plant-based milk of your choice)
- 1 teaspoon pure maple syrup or raw honey (optional for a touch of sweetness)
- ½ teaspoon pure vanilla extract

- Fresh berries and sliced almonds for topping

Instructions:

1. In a mason jar or airtight container, combine chia seeds, almond milk, maple syrup or raw honey (if using), and vanilla extract.

2. Stir well to ensure the chia seeds are evenly distributed.

3. Close the jar/container tightly and refrigerate overnight or for at least 4 hours. During this time, the chia seeds will absorb the liquid and form a delicious pudding-like texture.

4. Once the chia seed pudding has set, give it a good stir.

5. Top the pudding with fresh berries and sliced almonds for added flavor and crunch.

6. Enjoy your Alkaline Chia Seed Pudding as a refreshing and filling breakfast!

3.3 Zesty Citrus Avocado Toast

Ingredients:

- 2 slices of whole-grain or sprouted grain bread (gluten-free if desired)
- 1 ripe avocado, peeled and pitted
- Juice and zest of 1 organic lemon
- ½ teaspoon red pepper flakes (adjust to your spice preference)
- Sea salt and black pepper to taste
- Fresh cilantro leaves for garnish (optional)

Instructions:

1. Toast the slices of bread to your desired form of crispiness.

2. While the bread is toasting, scoop the ripe avocado into a bowl and mash it with a fork until smooth.

3. Add the lemon juice, lemon zest, red pepper flakes, sea salt, and black pepper to the mashed avocado. Stir well to mix all the flavors.

4. Once the bread is toasted, spread the zesty avocado mixture evenly onto each slice.

5. Garnish the avocado toast with fresh cilantro leaves for an extra burst of flavor (if using).

6. Serve the Zesty Citrus Avocado Toast immediately and savor the refreshing and tangy taste!

These energizing breakfast recipes for a healthy alkaline diet will not only help balance your pH levels but also provide your body with essential nutrients to kickstart your day on a positive note. Incorporating alkaline-rich foods into your morning routine can boost your energy levels, support digestion, and promote overall well-being. Enjoy these delicious and nutritious breakfast options for a healthful start to your day!

Chapter Four

Nutrient-Rich Lunchtime Delights

4.1 Rainbow Veggie Quinoa Salad

Ingredients:

- 1 cup tri-color quinoa, rinsed and cooked according to package instructions
- 1 cup cherry tomatoes, halved
- 1 cup cucumber, diced
- 1 cup shredded carrots
- 1 cup purple cabbage, finely sliced
- 1 cup baby spinach leaves
- 1/4 cup fresh parsley, chopped
- 1/4 cup fresh mint, chopped
- 1/4 cup roasted sunflower seeds
- 2 tablespoons extra-virgin olive oil
- 2 tablespoons lemon juice

- 1 tablespoon apple cider vinegar

- 1 teaspoon Dijon mustard

- Salt and pepper to taste

Instructions:

1. In a large mixing bowl, combine the cooked quinoa, cherry tomatoes, cucumber, shredded carrots, purple cabbage, baby spinach, parsley, and mint.

2. In a small bowl, mix the olive oil, lemon juice, apple cider vinegar, Dijon mustard, salt, and pepper until well combined.

3. Drizzle the dressing over the quinoa salad and toss gently to coat all the ingredients.

4. Sprinkle roasted sunflower seeds on top for added crunch and nutty flavor.

5. Serve the Rainbow Veggie Quinoa Salad chilled or at room temperature, and enjoy a vibrant medley of flavors and textures that will leave you feeling energized and satisfied.

4.2 Creamy Alkaline Gazpacho Soup

Ingredients:

- 4 large tomatoes, roughly chopped
- 1 medium cucumber, peeled and diced
- 1 small red bell pepper (seeded and chopped)
- 1 small green bell pepper (seeded and chopped)
- 1/2 small red onion, chopped
- 2 cloves garlic, minced
- 2 cups watermelon, diced
- 1/4 cup fresh basil leaves

- 2 tablespoons fresh lemon juice
- 1 tablespoon extra-virgin olive oil
- 1 teaspoon Himalayan salt
- 1/2 teaspoon ground black pepper
- Pinch of cayenne pepper (optional, for a subtle kick)
- Fresh basil leaves and diced cucumber for garnish

Instructions:

1. In a blender, combine the tomatoes, cucumber, red and green bell peppers, red onion, garlic, watermelon, and fresh basil.

2. Blend the ingredients until smooth and creamy.

3. Add the lemon juice, olive oil, Himalayan salt, black pepper, and cayenne pepper (if

using) to the blender and pulse briefly to incorporate the flavors.

4. Transfer the gazpacho soup to a large bowl, cover, and refrigerate for at least 30 minutes to let the flavors meld.

5. Before serving, garnish with fresh basil leaves and diced cucumber to add an extra burst of freshness and texture.

6. Indulge in this creamy alkaline gazpacho soup, bursting with antioxidants and hydrating properties, making it a perfect choice for a hot summer's day.

4.3 Mediterranean Stuffed Bell Peppers

Ingredients:

- 4 large bell peppers (assorted colors), tops removed and seeds removed
- 1 cup cooked quinoa (from 1/2 cup dry quinoa)
- 1 cup canned chickpeas (drained and rinsed)
- 1/2 cup crumbled feta cheese (omit for a vegan version or use a plant-based alternative)
- 1/4 cup black olives, sliced
- 1/4 cup sundried tomatoes, chopped
- 2 tablespoons fresh lemon juice
- 2 tablespoons chopped fresh oregano
- 1 tablespoon extra-virgin olive oil
- 2 cloves garlic, minced
- Salt and pepper to taste

Instructions:

1. Preheat your oven to 375°F (190°C). Place the prepared bell peppers in a baking dish and set aside.

2. In a mixing bowl, combine the cooked quinoa, chickpeas, crumbled feta cheese (if using), black olives, sun dried tomatoes, lemon juice, fresh oregano, olive oil, minced garlic, salt, and pepper.

3. Stuff each bell pepper with the quinoa mixture until they are generously filled.

4. Cover the baking dish with foil and bake the stuffed bell peppers for 25-30 minutes or until the peppers are tender.

5. Remove the foil and continue baking for an additional 5-7 minutes to lightly brown the tops.

6. Let the Mediterranean Stuffed Bell Peppers cool for a few minutes before serving.

7. Savor the Mediterranean flavors, complete with protein-rich chickpeas, whole grains, and aromatic herbs—a delightful combination of taste and nutrition.

Enjoy these creations, and may they bring you a fulfilling and wholesome lunchtime experience like no other!

Chapter Five

Nourishing Dinner Options

5.1 Baked Portobello Mushrooms with Garlic Kale

Ingredients:

- 4 large Portobello mushrooms
- 2 cups kale, chopped
- 4 cloves garlic, minced
- 1 tablespoon olive oil
- 2 tablespoons balsamic vinegar
- 1 teaspoon dried thyme
- Salt and pepper to taste
- Grated Parmesan cheese (optional)

Instructions:

1. Preheat your oven to 375°F (190°C) and lightly grease a baking sheet.

2. Clean the Portobello mushrooms using a damp cloth, removing any dirt or debris. Gently remove the stems and scrape out the gills using a spoon to create more room for the filling.

3. In a small bowl, mix olive oil, minced garlic, dried thyme, balsamic vinegar, salt, and pepper.

4. Brush the mixture generously onto both sides of the mushrooms, ensuring they are evenly coated.

5. Place the mushrooms on the prepared baking sheet, gill-side up, and bake for 15 minutes or until they become tender.

6. Meanwhile, in a large skillet, sauté the chopped kale with a little olive oil until it wilts and turns bright green. Season with a pinch of salt and pepper.

7. Once the mushrooms are done, fill each cap with the sautéed kale, pressing it down gently to fit more in.

8. Optionally, sprinkle some grated Parmesan cheese on top for added richness and flavor.

9. Return the stuffed mushrooms to the oven and bake for an additional 5-7 minutes, until the cheese melts (if using) and the kale is slightly crispy.

10. Serve hot and enjoy this delightful and nutritious dinner option!

5.2 Coconut Curry Lentil Stew

Ingredients:

- 1 cup dry red lentils, rinsed and drained
- 1 can (14 oz) coconut milk
- 2 cups vegetable broth
- 1 onion, finely chopped

- 2 carrots, diced
- 1 red bell pepper, chopped
- 3 cloves garlic, minced
- 1 tablespoon curry powder
- 1 teaspoon ground cumin
- 1 teaspoon ground turmeric
- 1 tablespoon vegetable oil
- Salt and pepper to taste
- Fresh cilantro for garnish
- Cooked rice or naan bread (optional, for serving)

Instructions:

1. Heat the vegetable oil in a large pot over medium heat. Add the chopped onion and sauté until it becomes translucent.

2. Stir in the minced garlic, curry powder, ground cumin, and ground turmeric. Cook for another minute until fragrant.

3. Add the diced carrots and red bell pepper to the pot. Cook for a few minutes until they start to soften.

4. Pour in the rinsed lentils and vegetable broth, stirring everything together.

5. Bring the mixture to a boil, then reduce the heat to a simmer. Cover the pot and let it cook for about 20-25 minutes or until the lentils are tender and the stew has thickened.

6. Stir in the coconut milk and let it simmer for an additional 5 minutes to meld the flavors together.

7. Season with salt and pepper to taste. If you prefer a spicier stew, you can add a pinch of red pepper flakes.

8. Serve the Coconut Curry Lentil Stew over a bed of fluffy rice or with some warm naan bread. Garnish with fresh cilantro for a burst of freshness.

5.3 Roasted Cauliflower Steaks with Tahini Dressing

Ingredients:

- 1 large head of cauliflower
- 2 tablespoons olive oil
- 1 teaspoon ground cumin
- 1 teaspoon smoked paprika
- 1/2 teaspoon garlic powder
- Salt and pepper to taste
- 2 tablespoons tahini
- 2 tablespoons water
- 1 tablespoon lemon juice
- 1 tablespoon maple syrup
- 1 clove garlic, minced
- 1 tablespoon chopped parsley (optional, for garnish)

Instructions:

1. Preheat your oven to 400°F (200°C) and line a baking sheet with parchment paper.

2. Remove the leaves and trim the stem of the cauliflower, making sure it stands upright. Carefully slice the cauliflower vertically into 3/4-inch thick steaks.

3. In a small bowl, mix olive oil, ground cumin, smoked paprika, garlic powder, salt, and pepper.

4. Brush both sides of each cauliflower steak with the spice mixture and place them on the prepared baking sheet.

5. Roast the cauliflower in the preheated oven for about 25 minutes or until tender and golden brown, flipping them halfway through for even roasting.

6. In the meantime, prepare the tahini dressing. In a bowl, whisk the tahini, water,

lemon juice, maple syrup, minced garlic, and a pinch of salt until smooth and creamy.

7. Once the cauliflower steaks are ready, transfer them to a serving platter and drizzle the tahini dressing over the top.

8. Optionally, garnish with chopped parsley for a burst of color and freshness.

9. Serve the Roasted Cauliflower Steaks with Tahini Dressing as a hearty and wholesome dinner option that's sure to impress!

Enjoy these nourishing dinner options, perfect for a satisfying and healthy meal with loved ones.

Chapter Six

Tasty Snacks to Satisfy Cravings

6.1 Alkaline Trail Mix

Ingredients:

- 1 cup almonds

- 1 cup walnuts

- 1 cup pumpkin seeds

- 1 cup dried goji berries

- 1 cup dried mulberries

- 1 tablespoon coconut oil

- 1 tablespoon maple syrup

- 1 teaspoon turmeric powder

- 1 teaspoon spirulina powder

- 1/2 teaspoon sea salt

Instructions:

1. Preheat the oven to 300°F (150°C) and line a baking sheet with parchment paper.

2. In a large mixing bowl, combine the almonds, walnuts, pumpkin seeds, dried goji berries, and dried mulberries.

3. In a saucepan, melt the coconut oil over low heat. After has melted, stir in the maple syrup, turmeric powder, spirulina powder, and sea salt. Stir well until properly combined.

4. Pour the liquid mixture over the nut and berry mixture, and toss well to coat all the ingredients evenly.

5. Spread the mixture in a single layer on the prepared baking sheet.

6. Bake in the preheated oven for 20-25 minutes, stirring halfway through to ensure even toasting.

7. Remove from the oven and let the trail mix cool completely before storing in an airtight container.

8. Enjoy this alkaline trail mix as a nutritious and satisfying snack on the go!

6.2 Baked Zucchini Chips with Cashew Dip

Ingredients:

For the zucchini chips:

- 2 large zucchinis, thinly sliced
- 1/4 cup almond flour
- 1/4 cup nutritional yeast
- 1 teaspoon garlic powder
- 1 teaspoon smoked paprika
- 1/2 teaspoon onion powder
- 1/2 teaspoon sea salt
- 1/4 teaspoon black pepper
- 2 tablespoons olive oil

For the cashew dip:

- 1 cup raw cashews, soaked in water for 4 hours or overnight
- 1/4 cup water
- 2 tablespoons lemon juice
- 1 tablespoon nutritional yeast
- 1 clove garlic
- 1/2 teaspoon sea salt
- Fresh parsley (for garnish)

Instructions:

1. Preheat the oven to 375°F (190°C), line a baking sheet with parchment paper.

2. In a shallow dish, combine almond flour, nutritional yeast, garlic powder, smoked paprika, onion powder, sea salt, and black pepper for the zucchini chips.

3. Dip each zucchini slice into the olive oil, making sure both sides are coated, then dredge it in the almond flour mixture, pressing gently to adhere the mixture to the zucchini.

4. Place the coated zucchini slices on the prepared baking sheet in a single layer, ensuring they do not overlap.

5. Bake in the preheated oven for 25-30 minutes or until the zucchini chips turn golden and crispy.

6. While the zucchini chips are baking, prepare the cashew dip. Drain the soaked cashews and place them in a blender or food processor.

7. Add water, lemon juice, nutritional yeast, garlic, and sea salt to the blender with the cashews. Blend until smooth and creamy. If

needed, add a bit more water to achieve the desired consistency.

8. Transfer the cashew dip to a serving bowl and garnish with chopped fresh parsley.

9. Serve the baked zucchini chips with the creamy cashew dip for a delicious and wholesome snack!

6.3 Refreshing Cucumber and Watermelon Salad

Ingredients:
- 2 cups diced cucumber
- 2 cups diced watermelon
- 1/4 cup crumbled feta cheese
- 1/4 cup fresh mint leaves, torn
- 2 tablespoons lime juice
- 1 tablespoon honey
- 1/4 teaspoon ground cumin
- Pinch of salt and black pepper

Instructions:

1. In a large mixing bowl, combine the diced cucumber and watermelon.

2. In a separate small bowl, whisk together the lime juice, honey, ground cumin, salt, and black pepper to create the dressing.

3. Pour the dressing over the cucumber and watermelon mixture, and gently toss to coat all the ingredients evenly.

4. Sprinkle the crumbled feta cheese and torn mint leaves over the salad, and give it a light toss.

5. Chill the cucumber and watermelon salad in the refrigerator for at least 15 minutes before serving to allow the flavors to meld together.

6. Serve this refreshing salad on a hot day or as a side dish to complement any meal. It's a delightful and hydrating treat!

Chapter Seven

Indulgent Desserts with a Healthy Twist

7.1 Decadent Almond Butter and Banana Nice Cream

Ingredients:

- 4 ripe bananas, peeled and sliced
- 1/2 cup almond butter (unsweetened and creamy)
- 1/4 cup almond milk (unsweetened)
- 1 tablespoon pure maple syrup
- 1 teaspoon pure vanilla extract
- A pinch of sea salt
- 2 tablespoons dark chocolate chips (optional, for topping)

Instructions:

1. In a blender or food processor, combine the sliced bananas, almond butter, almond milk, pure maple syrup, vanilla extract, and a pinch of sea salt.

2. Blend the ingredients until smooth and creamy, scraping down the sides if needed to ensure everything is well mixed.

3. Taste the mixture and adjust sweetness if desired by adding more maple syrup.

4. Once the mixture is smooth and well-combined, transfer it to a freezer-safe container, spreading it evenly.

5. If you prefer a touch of chocolate, sprinkle dark chocolate chips over the top of the nice cream.

6. Cover the container with a lid or reusable wrap, and place it in the freezer for at least 4 hours or until fully frozen.

7. When ready to serve, let the nice cream sit at room temperature for a few minutes to soften slightly, making it easier to scoop.

8. Enjoy this guilt-free indulgence with a healthy twist!

7.2 Raw Vegan Lemon Bars

Ingredients:

For the crust:

- 1 cup raw almonds
- 1/2 cup shredded coconut (unsweetened)
- 5-6 Medjool dates (pitted)
- Zest of 1 lemon

For the lemon filling:

- 1 cup raw cashews (soaked in water for at least 4 hours and drained)
- 1/4 cup coconut oil (melted)
- 1/4 cup fresh lemon juice

- 1/4 cup pure maple syrup

- Zest of 2 lemons

- 1 teaspoon pure vanilla extract

- A pinch of sea salt

Instructions:

1. Prepare an 8x8-inch baking dish by lining it with parchment paper, leaving some extra paper hanging over the sides for easy removal later.

2. In a food processor, combine the raw almonds, shredded coconut, pitted dates, and lemon zest for the crust. Pulse until the mixture resembles coarse crumbs and sticks together when pressed between your fingers.

3. Press the crust mixture firmly and evenly into the bottom of the prepared baking dish. Smooth it out with the back of a spoon.

4. In the same food processor (you don't need to clean it), put the soaked and drained cashews, melted coconut oil, fresh lemon juice, pure maple syrup, lemon zest, vanilla extract, and a pinch of sea salt inside and blend.

5. Blend the filling ingredients until smooth and creamy, scraping down the sides as needed to ensure there are no lumps.

6. Pour the lemon filling over the crust in the baking dish, spreading it out evenly.

7. Cover the dish with a lid or reusable wrap and place it in the refrigerator to set for at least 3 hours or until firm.

8. Once the lemon bars have set, lift them out of the baking dish using the parchment paper overhang, and place them on a cutting board.

9. Cut the bars into desired shapes and sizes using a sharp knife.

10. Serve these refreshing raw vegan lemon bars as a delightful and healthy treat!

7.3 Guilt-Free Chocolate Avocado Mousse

Ingredients:

- 2 ripe avocados, peeled and pitted
- 1/4 cup unsweetened cocoa powder
- 1/4 cup pure maple syrup
- 1/4 cup almond milk (unsweetened)
- 1 teaspoon pure vanilla extract
- A pinch of sea salt
- Fresh berries (such as raspberries or strawberries) for garnish

Instructions:

1. In a blender or food processor, combine the ripe avocados, unsweetened cocoa

powder, pure maple syrup, almond milk, pure vanilla extract, and a pinch of sea salt.

2. Blend the ingredients until smooth and creamy, making sure there are no avocado chunks left.

3. Taste the mousse and adjust sweetness if needed by adding more maple syrup.

4. Once the mousse is smooth and velvety, transfer it to serving bowls or glasses.

5. Cover the bowls or glasses with reusable wrap and refrigerate for at least 1 hour to chill and set the mousse.

6. Before serving, garnish each portion with fresh berries for a burst of flavor and an elegant touch.

7. Savor this guilt-free chocolate avocado mousse, knowing you're treating yourself to a delightful, nutrient-rich dessert!

Chapter Eight

Incorporating Superfoods into Your Alkaline Vegan Diet

8.1 Exploring the Power of Superfoods

Incorporating superfoods into your alkaline vegan diet can be a game-changer for your overall health and well-being. Superfoods are nutrient-dense foods that are packed with vitamins, minerals, antioxidants, and other essential compounds that can provide numerous health benefits. They are nature's powerhouse, offering an extraordinary array of nutrients that can support your body's functions and promote vitality.

From antioxidant-rich berries to nutrient-packed greens, superfoods play a crucial role in maintaining a balanced pH level in the body, supporting alkalinity, and ensuring optimal functioning of various bodily systems. By including these nutrient-dense marvels into your diet, you can experience a natural boost in energy levels, improved digestion, enhanced immune function, and even a glowing complexion.

8.2 Acai Berry Bowl with Alkaline Fruits

One delectable and visually enticing way to incorporate superfoods into your alkaline vegan diet is through an Acai Berry Bowl with alkaline fruits. The star of this dish is the acai berry, renowned for its exceptional antioxidant content, promoting heart health and reducing inflammation. Combining it with a selection of alkaline fruits further enhances its benefits and flavors.

Start by blending frozen acai berries with ripe bananas and a splash of plant-based milk to achieve a thick and creamy consistency. Pour the vibrant purple mixture into a bowl, and now comes the fun part - topping it with an assortment of alkaline fruits. Slices of fresh kiwi, juicy chunks of watermelon, and a handful of antioxidant-rich blueberries can create a burst of colors and flavors that delight the taste buds.

For an added nutritional punch, sprinkle chia seeds or flaxseeds over the top. These seeds are rich in omega-3 fatty acids, fiber, and protein, further supporting your alkaline vegan lifestyle. With each spoonful, you'll not only experience a symphony of textures and tastes but also nourish your body with a bounty of nutrients.

8.3   Spirulina-infused   Green Smoothie

Another fantastic way to infuse your alkaline vegan diet with superfoods is by blending up a Spirulina-infused Green Smoothie. Spirulina, a blue-green algae, is a nutritional powerhouse, loaded with essential vitamins, minerals, and plant-based protein. Adding it to your green smoothie can give your body a fantastic boost of nutrients while maintaining the alkalinity crucial for overall health.

To create this invigorating concoction, blend together a handful of alkaline greens like spinach, kale, and cucumber with a ripe banana for natural sweetness. Add a generous scoop of spirulina powder and a splash of coconut water or almond milk for a smooth consistency.

The resulting vibrant green smoothie is not only visually appealing but also a nutrient-packed elixir. Sip on this goodness, and you'll be flooding your body with chlorophyll, iron, vitamin C, and other potent antioxidants, which can support detoxification and boost your immune system.

Remember, the key to a successful alkaline vegan lifestyle lies in variety and balance. Explore the diverse range of superfoods available, experiment with new recipes, and always listen to your body's needs. With time, you'll discover the incredible benefits of these nutrient-dense wonders, and your body will thank you for making such nourishing choices. So, embrace the power of superfoods and embark on a path to a healthier and more vibrant you.

Chapter Nine

Hydration and Detoxification

In recent years, the significance of maintaining a healthy lifestyle has gained immense popularity. Among the various aspects that contribute to overall well-being, hydration and detoxification stand out as crucial components. In this chapter, we will explore the importance of staying hydrated on an alkaline vegan diet, and delve into the benefits of two refreshing detox drinks - Lemon Ginger Water and Cucumber and Mint Detox Drink.

9.1 Importance of Hydration on an Alkaline Vegan Diet

Hydration plays a pivotal role in sustaining an alkaline vegan diet. This dietary approach emphasizes the consumption of whole, plant-based foods that contribute to a more alkaline pH in the body. However, even with a balanced vegan diet, neglecting proper hydration can hinder the body's ability to maintain its pH balance.

Water is vital for various bodily functions, including digestion, nutrient absorption, and waste elimination. When following an alkaline vegan diet, the body needs to neutralize acidic byproducts from metabolism and digestion. Ample water intake aids in flushing out toxins and maintaining the body's pH levels within the optimal range, which is crucial for overall health and well-being.

To ensure adequate hydration, individuals on an alkaline vegan diet should aim to drink at least 8 to 10 cups of water daily, in addition to obtaining water from hydrating fruits and vegetables. By staying well-hydrated, one can maximize the benefits of an alkaline vegan diet and promote a harmonious internal environment.

9.2 Detoxifying Lemon Ginger Water

Lemon Ginger Water stands out as an excellent detoxifying beverage that complements an alkaline vegan diet. This simple yet powerful concoction combines the cleansing properties of lemon and ginger, creating a refreshing drink that aids in detoxification and hydration.

Lemons are rich in vitamin C, a potent antioxidant that supports the immune system and helps neutralize free radicals in the body. Additionally, lemons possess natural diuretic properties, promoting the elimination of waste and toxins through urine.

Ginger, on the other hand, is well-known for its anti-inflammatory and digestive benefits. It stimulates the digestive system, helps alleviate bloating, and can even aid in weight management. Ginger also contains antioxidants that assist in detoxifying the body and reducing oxidative stress.

To prepare Lemon Ginger Water, simply slice a fresh lemon and a piece of ginger, and add them to a jug of water. Allow the ingredients to infuse for a few hours or overnight in the refrigerator. Regular consumption of this revitalizing drink can contribute to enhanced detoxification and hydration, promoting overall health and vitality.

9.3 Refreshing Cucumber and Mint Detox Drink

Another fantastic option for detoxification and hydration is the Cucumber and Mint Detox Drink. Cucumbers are renowned for their high water content, making them naturally hydrating and beneficial for flushing out toxins. They are also a good source of vitamins and minerals, further enhancing the nutritional value of this detox drink.

Mint leaves not only add a refreshing flavor but also provide numerous health benefits. Mint has been traditionally used to soothe digestive issues, alleviate bloating, and promote healthy skin. Moreover, it aids in the body's natural detoxification processes by supporting liver function, a vital organ responsible for filtering and eliminating toxins.

To create this delicious detox drink, thinly slice a cucumber and add a handful of fresh mint leaves to a pitcher of water. Allow the mixture to infuse for a few hours before enjoying its refreshing taste and rejuvenating effects.

Hydration and detoxification play integral roles in maintaining a healthy and balanced lifestyle, especially on an alkaline vegan diet. Adequate water intake supports the body's pH balance and ensures optimal functioning of various bodily processes. Incorporating detoxifying drinks like Lemon Ginger Water and Cucumber and Mint Detox Drink can further enhance the benefits of proper hydration, helping to rid the body of harmful toxins and promoting overall well-being. By prioritizing hydration and embracing these refreshing detox drinks, individuals can take a proactive step towards a healthier, more vibrant life on their alkaline vegan journey.

Chapter Ten

Creating Balance and Sustainable Habits

Maintaining a balanced and sustainable lifestyle is essential for overall well-being. In recent years, the alkaline vegan diet has gained popularity for its potential health benefits. However, achieving long-term success with this dietary choice requires integrating it with other lifestyle factors and staying motivated on the healing journey. Here, you will explore how to strike a harmonious balance between an alkaline vegan diet and other aspects of life, offering valuable tips for long-term success and ways to stay motivated throughout the transformational process.

10.1 Balancing Alkaline Vegan Diet with Other Lifestyle Factors

While the alkaline vegan diet is centered around consuming whole, plant-based foods that promote an alkaline pH in the body, it is crucial to consider other aspects of life that influence overall health. Some essential tips for finding balance are:

1. **Regular Exercise:** Physical activity is vital for a balanced lifestyle. Engage in activities you enjoy, such as walking, jogging, yoga, or dancing. Exercise not only supports your overall well-being but also helps maintain a healthy body weight.

2. **Hydration:** Drink plenty water throughout the day, this way you'll be hydrated all through the day. Hydration is

important for taking out toxins and maintaining proper bodily functions.

3. **Stress Management:** Chronic stress can negatively impact health. Incorporate relaxation techniques like meditation, deep breathing, or spending time in nature to reduce stress levels.

4. **Social Connections:** Cultivate strong social bonds with family and friends. Positive relationships can improve mental and emotional well-being.

5. **Adequate Sleep:** Aim for 7-9 hours of quality sleep per night. Sufficient rest is crucial for the body to rejuvenate and repair itself.

10.2 Tips for Long-term Success

Creating sustainable habits with an alkaline vegan lifestyle can lead to long-term success. These are tips you should follow to make the journey smoother:

1. **Gradual Transition:** Shift to an alkaline vegan diet gradually. Allow your body and taste buds to adapt to the changes over time. Sudden, drastic changes may lead to frustration and setbacks.

2. **Nutritional Variety:** Ensure you are consuming a diverse range of alkaline foods to obtain a wide spectrum of nutrients. Be sure to have fruits, vegetables, whole grains, nuts, and seeds in your diet.

3. **Meal Planning:** Plan your meals ahead to avoid resorting to unhealthy options when hungry. This practice can also help you stay on track with your dietary goals.

4. **Seek Support:** Join online communities or local groups that share similar dietary interests. Surrounding yourself with like-minded individuals can provide encouragement and inspiration.

5. **Regular Check-ins:** Monitor your progress and make adjustments as needed. Celebrate your achievements, no matter how small, to stay motivated.

10.3 Staying Motivated on Your Healing Journey

Maintaining motivation throughout your healing journey is crucial to achieving long-term success. Stay motivated following these strategies:

1. **Set True Goals:** Establish achievable short-term and long-term goals. Celebrate your accomplishments along the way, which will keep you motivated to reach bigger milestones.

2. **Journaling:** Keep a journal to track your progress, emotions, and reflections. This practice can help you stay accountable and gain insights into your journey.

3. **Visualize Success:** Imagine yourself leading a balanced and vibrant life. Visualization can reinforce your commitment to the healing process.

4. **Continuous Learning:** Stay informed about the alkaline vegan diet and its benefits. Understanding the science behind it can provide motivation and reassurance.

5. **Embrace Imperfection:** Acknowledge that setbacks are a natural part of any journey. Be kind to yourself and use challenges as opportunities for growth.

Creating balance and sustainable habits with an alkaline vegan lifestyle requires careful consideration of various lifestyle factors. By incorporating regular exercise, managing stress, and nurturing social connections, you can complement the benefits of an alkaline vegan diet. Moreover, long-term success can be achieved by adopting gradual changes, seeking support, and monitoring your progress. Stay motivated throughout your healing journey by setting realistic goals, keeping track of your experiences, and visualizing a healthier, happier version of yourself. Embrace the transformational process with patience and self-compassion, and the rewards of a balanced and sustainable lifestyle will be within your reach.

Embracing the Alkaline Vegan Healing Diet for Life

The Alkaline Vegan Healing Diet has emerged as a powerful and transformative lifestyle choice, offering numerous health benefits that extend far beyond the realms of traditional diets. Throughout this book, we have delved into the profound impacts of this plant-based approach to nourishment. From alkalizing the body's pH to fostering cellular rejuvenation, this diet offers a holistic path towards optimal well-being and a sustainable future.

One of the most striking revelations is the undeniable link between the foods we consume and our overall health. The Alkaline Vegan Healing Diet has revealed itself as a guiding light, showing that food can be both your medicine and your poison. By embracing whole, plant-based foods and eliminating acidic, processed items, you can unlock your body's innate healing potential and attain vibrant health.

The importance of an alkaline state within the body cannot be overstated. With the modern diet often teeming with acidic foods, it is little wonder that chronic illnesses, such as obesity, diabetes, and cardiovascular diseases, are on the rise. The Alkaline Vegan Healing Diet offers a way to combat these issues, reducing inflammation and creating an internal environment where diseases struggle to thrive.

Beyond physical health, this diet extends its reach to encompass mental and emotional well-being. The connection between gut health and mental health is well-established, and the alkaline vegan approach nourishes the gut microbiome, leading to improved mood, clarity of thought, and reduced anxiety and depression. The elimination of harmful substances commonly found in processed foods further contributes to a sense of mental clarity and focus.

Embracing this lifestyle has a positive impact on the environment. By reducing the consumption of animal products and opting for plant-based alternatives, individuals can significantly reduce their carbon footprint. The Alkaline Vegan Healing Diet aligns with the principles of sustainable living, making it a responsible choice for those concerned about the planet's future.

Although adopting this diet requires commitment and a willingness to explore new culinary horizons, the rewards are profound and far-reaching.

However, it is essential to acknowledge that each individual's journey towards embracing the Alkaline Vegan Healing Diet may be unique. Humans are different, and what works for one may not completely work for another. It is crucial to approach this lifestyle with an open mind and a willingness to adapt, allowing for personalized adjustments to meet one's specific nutritional needs and preferences.

As with any diet or lifestyle change, it is wise to seek guidance from healthcare professionals or nutritionists who are well-versed in plant-based nutrition. They can help individuals ensure that they are meeting their dietary requirements, including essential nutrients like vitamin B12, iron, and omega-3 fatty acids, which can sometimes be challenging to obtain solely from plant-based sources.

Embrace the power of food as medicine, not just for your own well-being but for the betterment of the planet and all its inhabitants. Together, as a global community, we have the potential to create a sustainable, thriving world—one alkaline vegan meal at a time.

BONUS

Alkaline Vegan Healing Food List

Here, you will find a comprehensive list of alkaline vegan foods that promote natural weight loss, enhance the immune system, and contribute to overall well-being. Emphasizing these nutrient-dense and health-boosting foods will assist you as a beginner in adopting an Alkaline Vegan Healing Diet with ease and confidence. Incorporating these foods into your daily meals will support your body's natural healing processes and foster a sustainable and healthy lifestyle.

1. Vegetables:
- Leafy greens
- Cruciferous vegetables
- Cucumbers

- Bell peppers (red, yellow, green)
- Zucchini
- Carrots
- Tomatoes
- Eggplant
- Asparagus
- Celery

2. Fruits:
- Lemons
- Limes
- Avocado
- Berries (strawberries, blueberries, raspberries, blackberries)
- Apples
- Pears
- Watermelon
- Cantaloupe
- Mangoes

- Pineapple
- Papaya
- Oranges

3. Whole Grains:

- Quinoa
- Brown rice
- Amaranth
- Buckwheat
- Millet

4. Legumes:

- Lentils
- Chickpeas (garbanzo beans)
- Black beans
- Kidney beans
- Mung beans
- Pinto beans

5. Nuts and Seeds:

- Almonds

- Walnuts

- Flaxseeds

- Chia seeds

- Hemp seeds

- Pumpkin seeds

- Sunflower seeds

6. Healthy Fats and Oils:

- Extra-virgin olive oil

- Coconut oil

- Avocado oil

7. Herbs and Spices:

- Turmeric

- Ginger

- Garlic

- Basil

- Cilantro (coriander)
- Parsley
- Rosemary
- Thyme
- Oregano
- Cumin
- Paprika
- Cayenne pepper
- Black pepper
- Sea salt (in moderation)

8. Beverages:
- Herbal teas (chamomile, peppermint, ginger)
- Freshly squeezed vegetable and fruit juices
- Alkaline water

9. Sweeteners (in moderation):
- Pure maple syrup

- Coconut nectar
- Stevia

10. Superfoods (optional but beneficial):
- Spirulina
- Chlorella
- Wheatgrass
- Maca powder
- Acai berries

Remember, the key to an Alkaline Vegan Healing Diet is to focus on whole, natural, and unprocessed foods while avoiding highly acidic and processed foods. This food list is a great starting point to inspire your meal planning and encourage a balanced, nourishing, and healing approach to eating. As you progress on your journey, you can experiment with various combinations and recipes to discover what works best for your body and health goals.

28-day meal plan for the Alkaline Vegan Healing Diet:

Week 1

Day 1

- Breakfast: Alkaline Green Smoothie (spinach, kale, cucumber, banana, and almond milk)
- Lunch: Quinoa Salad with Avocado, Cucumber, and Lemon Dressing
- Snack: Almonds and apple slices
- Dinner: Baked Portobello Mushrooms with Garlic and Thyme, served with Steamed Broccoli

Day 2

- Breakfast: Chia Seed Pudding together with Fresh Berries

- Lunch: Zucchini Noodles with Tomato-Basil Sauce
- Snack: Carrot sticks with hummus
- Dinner: Lentil and Vegetable Stew with a side of Mixed Greens Salad

Day 3

- Breakfast: Overnight Oats with Almond Milk, Chopped Nuts, and Sliced Banana
- Lunch: Roasted Cauliflower and Chickpea Salad
- Snack: Sliced cucumbers with tahini
- Dinner: Stuffed Bell Peppers with Quinoa and Black Beans

Day 4

- Breakfast: Acai Bowl with Almond Butter and Granola
- Lunch: Spinach and Kale Salad with Chickpeas, Avocado, and Lemon-Tahini Dressing

- Snack: Mixed Berries
- Dinner: Baked Sweet Potato with Grilled Asparagus and Lemon-Garlic Sauce

Day 5

- Breakfast: Green Smoothie Bowl (avocado, spinach, mango, and coconut water)
- Lunch: Collard Wraps with Hummus, Shredded Carrots, Cucumber, and Sprouts
- Snack: Rice cakes with almond butter
- Dinner: Cauliflower Rice Stir-Fry with Tofu and Mixed Vegetables

Day 6

- Breakfast: Coconut Yogurt Parfait with Fresh Fruit and Hemp Seeds
- Lunch: Quinoa and Lentil Stuffed Bell Peppers
- Snack: Sliced Bell Peppers with Guacamole

- Dinner: Grilled Eggplant with Tomato Sauce and Basil, served with a side of Steamed Brussels Sprouts

Day 7

- Breakfast: Smoothie with Almond Milk, Banana, Blueberries, and a handful of Spinach
- Lunch: Raw Zucchini Noodles with Pesto and Cherry Tomatoes
- Snack: Orange slices
- Dinner: Baked Portobello Mushrooms with Mashed Cauliflower and Garlic

Week 2, 3, and 4

(Note: Repeat meals from Week 1 or feel free to create variations using similar ingredients.)

It is important to drink plenty of water throughout the day and adjust portion sizes according to your individual needs and activity level. It's also a good idea to include herbal teas and infusions for added variety and health benefits.

Before making significant changes to your diet, consult with a qualified healthcare professional or registered dietitian to ensure it aligns with your individual health needs and medical conditions.

Enjoy your journey with the Alkaline Vegan Healing Diet and make sure to combine it with regular exercise and a healthy lifestyle for optimal results.

Happy and Healthy Cooking!